ANCHOR TO YOUR STRENGTHS

ANCHOR TO YOUR STRENGTHS

Combining the Science of Who You Are
with the Chemistry of Essential Oils

MELINDA J. BRECHEISEN

DISCLAIMER

The information contained in this book has not been evaluated or approved by the US Food and Drug Administration or any other regulatory agency. The contents do not intend to diagnose, treat, cure, or prevent disease. The information is for educational purposes only.

The author of this book has expressed good-faith opinions and does not have or imply to have any professional medical training or licensing. The author expressly disclaims any liability from the use of the information contained in this book or from any adverse outcome resulting from the use of the information contained herein for any reason. In no event shall the authors of this book be liable for any direct, indirect, consequential, special, exemplary, or other damages related to the use of the information contained in this book. Consult a medical professional before using an herbal supplement or natural product.

The author of this book is not employed by, affiliated with, or sponsored by Gallup®. Opinions, views, and interpretations of CliftonStrengths® contained herein are the sole belief of the author.

ISBN: 1548660515
ISBN 13: 9781548660512
Library of Congress Control Number:2017916314
CreateSpace Independent Publishing Platform, North Charles

To my husband, Jeremie:

Thank you for believing in me.

And to my three children, Eliza, Aislin, and Oliver:
You are my sunshine and my joy.

Love, Melinda

CONTENTS

ACKNOWLEDGMENTS

Thank you, Drs. Bill and Lauren Moss, for the brainstorming session that created this idea.

Thank you, Laura and Jerry Jacobs, for inviting me to the table and giving me access to your team of brilliant minds.

Thank you, Bryan Terry, for your keen eye.

Thank you, Paul Allen, for your support.

To Eileen Engelman, thank you for the design work, but also the advice along the way.

And Misty Silva, thank you for making sure we looked good.

Thank you to all my colleagues and friends who offered feedback throughout the process, with an extra nod to P. J. Hanks.

I would also like to thank Gallup® for their support in the writing of this book.

A QUICK NOTE BEFORE WE GET STARTED

CliftonStrengths® is one of the most tested and trusted assessments available for understanding who you are and what you do best.

My assumption is that if you are reading this book, you have taken CliftonStrengths® and have your results in hand. If you have not taken the assessment, stop now, place this book on the coffee table, take a stroll to your computer, and take the assessment. Give yourself about thirty minutes to complete it. My bit of advice is to take it without a lot of preparation. Go now. Go with your instincts. Respond quickly. Answer with what you *really* do, not with what you *wish* you did or think you should do. Be honest. You'll find the assessment online at the Gallup® Strengths Center.

Now, grab your top five results, and keep reading.

CHAPTER ONE:
DISCOVERING
MY
STRENGTHS

※   ※   ※

I can still remember what it felt like as I eagerly checked the results of my CliftonStrengths® talent assessment. It was a bit like biting into a fortune cookie and thinking that little slip of paper hiding inside would change my life, but with much higher expectations. In the next few moments, I would have my top five, the big five, the five words that would change everything. I knew it was going to be big—otherwise, Gallup® wouldn't use words like *undecillion* when describing just how unique and special I really was. I was very excited. And then, once I started reading, I was a bit confused.

Harmony®. That's an odd name for a strength, I thought. I began reading the description. And my heart fell. I hated it. I hated Harmony®. Harmony® sounded like the strength of a yellow-bellied coward. Harmony® sounded like the last person to be picked for the team. Harmony® sounded spineless. I quickly moved on down the list, thinking perhaps it was a mistake and the rest of my list would make sense.

Learner®. Check.

Relator®. Check.

Input®. I had no idea what that was, but at least it sounded smart, so I moved on.

And the final strength in my top five was Responsibility®. Check.

I took a second glance at Input® and connected with the description. I scrolled through the rest of my top five and decided that strengths two through five were a perfect match. So how could my number-one strength be so wrong?

Perhaps you can relate to my experience. Did you initially feel some resistance to identifying with and claiming your top five? Did it feel a little bit too much like a fortune cookie…like maybe it could have applied to anyone?

It isn't uncommon to struggle when first understanding your talents. In fact, culturally, we spend very little time trying to understand our talents, and instead we invest our time in areas we think need improvement. All you need to do is ask a room of people to tell you five great things about themselves to see just how uncomfortable we are with talking about what is right within ourselves. I felt such resistance to my talent assessment that I sought out coaching from a certified Gallup® Strengths Coach.

Through coaching, I was able to unravel my strengths. Not only did I realize that Harmony® was, indeed, my number one strength, but I was also able to recognize its driving force in every major decision I had ever made. And most importantly, I was able to recognize that while it influenced my life in profound ways, it was not always being used for good. It was a bit like rolling the dice. Maybe it would be used productively. Maybe it wouldn't. Maybe it would show up when it was advantageous. Maybe it would be missing in action during a crucial conversation. It was easy to see that Harmony® was a powerful force in my life, but I wasn't the one in charge. It made sense that my response to Harmony® was one of repulsion. Harmony® was the boss of me. And I resented it.

The intent of this book is to present a method for gaining control of your strengths. If you can learn to turn them on and off, you can set yourself up for success. Woo® (winning others over) is an amazing strength when you need to attend a party full of strangers. But Woo® may not be the first strength you want to tap into at a funeral. Deliberative® is an amazing strength when you want to make a solid decision and move confidently forward. Deliberative® may not be that great if it results in the inability to make a decision at all.

By anchoring your strengths, you are empowered. You are in the driver's seat. Anchoring is an investment in your strengths that allows you to wield your strengths at will. By learning how to use your strengths intentionally, you can turn moments of opportunity into moments of success.

CHAPTER TWO:
START WITH TALENT, END WITH STRENGTH

CliftonStrengths® is an assessment of normal personality for discovering who you are and what you do best. The assessment measures the presence of thirty-four areas, or themes, and ranks them in order of dominance. These themes, referred to as talents, are the areas that we can develop and turn into strengths.

The CliftonStrengths® assessment is one of the most tested and trusted generalizable psychometric assessments in the world. According to Gallup's technical report, the assessment has been validated extensively, including test-retest reliability, contrast validity, and business-impact analyses. The assessment is extremely reliable.

Gallup® recently completed a meta-analysis of 2.1 million individuals who had taken the CliftonStrengths® assessment, spread across forty-nine thousand business units and forty-five countries. Here are a few of the results from this international study:

Customer Engagement: 3.4–6.9 percent increase

Employee Engagement: 9.0–15.0 percent increase

Profit: 14.4–29.4 percent increase

Safety Incidents: 22.0–59.0 percent decrease

Sales: 10.3–19.3 percent increase

Low Turnover Orgs: 5.8–16.1 points decrease in turnover

High Turnover Orgs: 26.0–71.8 points decrease in turnover

(Asplund et al. 2015)

Notice the ranges of impact. For some, knowing their strengths made a small difference, but for others the impact was significant. This is why knowing "what's next" and taking action with your strengths is so critical.

Gallup® also found that those who said they were able to use their strengths every day were three times more likely to rate the quality of their lives as excellent and six times more likely to be engaged.

The more you grow your strengths, the better your results in business and the higher your quality of life. It is well worth your time and investment to develop your talents into strengths.

By identifying talents and developing them into strengths, you can learn to work with others with more engagement and less conflict. You can learn how you make decisions and set yourself up for success by creating the environment that serves you best. You can spend more time in areas that create energy and clearly identify the areas best delegated to others. You can create a support team that balances and completes your strengths' domains by identifying blind spots and limitations within yourself and your team. You can create a common language among family, friends, colleagues, and associates that allows for open discussion, concise action planning, and forward movement.

CliftonStrengths® isn't a fortune cookie or a horoscope. It is an assessment that is developmental in nature. It is designed with the expectation that you will invest in your talents and begin to use your strengths constructively and consistently. Partnering your strengths with anchoring, a form of classical behavior conditioning, puts you in the driver's seat. By utilizing the sense of smell, the human body's most powerful sense, you create established connections, or anchors, that take strengths to the next level.

CHAPTER THREE:
WHAT ARE
ESSENTIAL OILS?

Essential oils are the naturally occurring volatile compounds found in plants. These oils are found in the plant material such as roots, stems, bark, seeds, and leaves. Through cold pressing or steam distillation, the essential oil is extracted from the plant material. The result is a very powerful, very concentrated aromatic compound.

There are more than three thousand varieties of volatile compounds found in essential oils. While essential oils have been used for hundreds of years for food preparation, perfumes, and rituals, it is through the scientific study of these volatile compounds that the modern application of essential oils for therapeutic benefit has emerged.

Not all essential oil brands are created equally. There is little to no regulation of the essential oils being sold on the market. When selecting essential oils for anchoring, quality is paramount. Take the time to research the brand you select.

Here are a few points to consider when choosing essential oils:

1. therapeutic grade or better
2. disclosure of sourcing and country of origin
3. GC/MS testing results for the bottle batch readily available
4. resources for education and product information available
5. tested and trusted

HOW TO USE ESSENTIAL OILS AND SAFETY

There are three methods of use for essential oils: aromatic, topical, and internal.

AROMATIC

Aromatic use simply means to inhale the oil. Opening the bottle and taking a nice deep breath is sufficient to receive the benefits of the oil. You can also place a drop in your hands and inhale by cupping your hands around your nose. You may also consider a diffuser. Diffusers allow you to affect a larger area, such as an office space or bedroom, by dispersing oil through the air.

TOPICAL

Topical use of essential oils refers to applying the essential oil directly to the skin. They are absorbed quickly and enter the bloodstream. Always dilute your oils before applying them to the skin. Dilute an essential oil with a carrier oil. A carrier oil is a lipid-based oil that helps with application and prevents rapid evaporation. Common carrier oils include coconut oil, extra virgin olive oil, jojoba oil, **grape-seed** oil, and almond oil.

INTERNAL

Internal use of essential oils involves taking the oils orally or sublingually. For anchoring, there is no need to use oils internally. Be sure to check for safety before using an oil internally, as not all brands are appropriate for this type of use.

SOME SAFETY TIPS

If you purchase a good-quality oil, it will arrive pure and concentrated. This extends the shelf life and allows for proper dilution based on need. When trying an oil for the first time, take a few drops of the carrier oil and one drop of the essential oil and apply to the bottom of your feet. As you get more comfortable with using oils, you can begin to use the oils on the back of your neck, wrists, and other areas. For anchoring purposes, you can usually simply smell the oil from the opened bottle or place one drop of essential oil in your hands and deeply inhale. However, for ease of application, you may want to make prediluted bottles of your favorite oils and keep them handy. To make a prediluted bottle purchase a ten-milliliter glass roll-on bottle, drop in ten drops of essential oil, and top off the remainder of the bottle with fractionated coconut oil. I have my oils in five-eighths dram bottles in a keychain, so they are instantly accessible. And lastly, do your research, use common sense, and trust your gut.

Keep oils out of reach of children and pets.

If you get oil in your eyes or experience skin irritation, use your carrier oil to dilute and wipe gently with a cloth. In a pinch, milk also works. Water is not recommended for this use.

CHAPTER FOUR:
ANCHORING

■ ■ ■

Anchoring is a powerful technique for controlling thoughts and emotions. As you anchor, you can choose your state of mind. By being able to instantaneously create a mind state, you can draw upon your strengths at will, allowing you to be at your best in the moments that matter.

Anchoring involves associating an emotional or physical state to an outside sensation. Typically, anchoring is done through sight, sound, or touch. You may be familiar with NLP (Neuro Linguistic Programming created by Richard Bandler and John Grinder) or EFT (Emotional Freedom Techniques created by Dr. Roger Callahan) which are both forms of anchoring. Tapping is anchoring with touch. Another common form of anchoring is affirmations. Affirmations are specific words you speak out loud to yourself to create specific results. Anchoring is a form of classical conditioning. Classical conditioning, in basic terms, means an association can trigger a response without conscious choice. The most famous example of classical conditioning was demonstrated by Ivan Pavlov and his famous dogs. Through experimentation, Pavlov recognized that the dogs salivated prior to consuming food. He rang a bell when the food was given to the dogs. Over time, the dogs would salivate to the ring of the bell with or without food present. The dogs were conditioned to respond to the bell without conscious choice.

Anchoring is a common practice among self-development experts like Tony Robbins. Anchoring is also used by professional athletes and entertainers. Many people use anchoring to increase performance and, more importantly, to create near-perfect performance again and again.

Smell is often overlooked and underappreciated as one of the senses. Humans can discriminate a few million colors and about a half a million tones. But we can discriminate *one trillion* olfactory stimuli. Because smell is in fact the most powerful of all the senses and provides a direct connection to the limbic brain, aromatic anchoring can be one of the most effective methods of classical conditioning.

Have you ever smelled someone's perfume or cologne and been immediately transported back in time? Reminiscing over a past lover or perhaps the smell of Grandma's couch? Ever walked into a home and the smell wafting from the kitchen brought you back to "that one summer you spent at the cabin"? These are examples of involuntary anchoring. Certain smells can trigger powerful memories and emotions. These moments happen to us all the time. They happen instantly without will or conscious thought. Imagine, then, if you could control it? When we *choose* to anchor a scent to a mind state, we can become intentional and take charge of our productivity and success at work and in relationships.

HOW DOES AROMATIC ANCHORING WORK?

We are creating a psychological association using our limbic brain by way of the olfactory system (as with Pavlov's dogs).

During inhalation, aromatic compounds travel through the nose and connect at receptor sites. These receptor sites send an immediate message to the olfactory bulb. The olfactory bulb is connected to the amygdala, hippocampus, and other parts of the brain. These sections of the brain are known as the "emotional brain," because they regulate memories, emotions, motivation, stress levels, and hormone balance. They also control the most primitive senses, such as basic drives, sexual arousal, and instincts.

Thus, by tapping into this part of the brain by way of inhalation of aromatic compounds, we can create powerful emotions and memories and draw upon those established connections at will.

CHAPTER FIVE:
HOW TO ANCHOR AN ESSENTIAL OIL

■ ▦ ▨

1. Choose the CliftonStrength® you want to anchor.

2. Choose the essential oil you want to anchor by looking at the three recommendations listed under the strength or by looking at the Quick-Reference Chart in the appendix. Make sure you choose a unique oil for each strength.

3. Think back to a time when you used that strength successfully. Imagine the state of mind. Imagine the energy being created. Consider the body language and words you used. If you need assistance, read the CliftonStrengths® Theme Description to guide you.

4. Take a drop of the essential oil and place it in your hand. Rub your hands together. Cup your hands over your nose, and inhale deeply, making sure you do not get the oil in your eyes. Safety note: if it's your first time trying a particular oil, dilute it with a carrier oil. Read your bottle to see if it can be used neat (undiluted) or if it needs a carrier oil.

5. As you deeply inhale the essential oil, play back the strength in your mind. Choose powerful language to describe the strength. Read the CliftonStrengths® Theme Description. Recall the powerful examples you have of when you used the strength successfully in the past.

6. Release your hands from your face and release your thoughts simultaneously. Shake your hands at your sides and allow your mind to wander.

7. Repeat this process several times, each time evoking powerful emotion and imagery as you inhale and anchor to your strength. You may need to reapply the essential oil if you feel the scent has faded.

8. Repeat this process in real time. When you are in a situation and you recognize you are using one strength predominantly, take out your essential oil and inhale to immediately connect it to your success.

9. Confirm the anchor. Take the essential oil in your hands and deeply inhale. See if you begin to feel the thoughts and emotions associated with the given strength. The thought process should happen within moments. If the response is not powerful enough of an association, you will need to anchor again throughout the week.

10. Recheck the anchor. Make sure it is permanent. The connection should feel the same every time.

11. If you do not have the experience you desire, do not continue to smell the essential oil. If you begin to feel frustrated or anxious, immediately break the thought pattern and remove your hands from your face. You do not want to anchor to a negative association.

12. Continue to reinforce the anchor by practicing and using the essential oil in situations where you successfully use the strength.

13. Repeat with each strength you wish to anchor. Make sure you use a unique oil for each strength.

14. Make your own essential oil blends using the strength recipes in chapter 9 to tap into your strengths throughout the day.

CHAPTER SIX:
THE CLIFTONSTRENGTHS®
INDEX

⬛   ⬛   ⬛

The following section contains the list of Gallup's thirty-four CliftonStrengths®, with their accompanying theme descriptions and essential oil suggestions. Each strength is described by its unique characteristics. These definitions are the official proprietary descriptions of Gallup, Inc. (Copyright © 2007 Gallup, Inc. Used here by express permission of Gallup, Inc. All rights reserved.)

Here is some suggested reading if you wish to study your strengths further:

Tom Rath, *Strength Finder 2.0*, Gallup®.

Tom Rath, *Strengths Based Leadership*, Gallup®.

Mary Reckmeyer, PhD, and Jennifer Robison, *Strengths Based Parenting*, Gallup®.

Through careful selection, I have paired each strength with an essential oil that promotes the use of that strength on a chemical level. I selected oils based on their physiological effect on the body and mind as discovered through scientific research. Many hours were spent poring over studies in the creation of this list. It is far from random. By looking at the chemical constituents of oils, we can decipher how the body will respond and choose oils accordingly.

For each strength, there are three oils to choose from. The first oil is the best option for that strength. However, because you do not want to anchor the same oil to more than one strength, each strength is given three options to avoid overlap. If you are already using the first option for another strength, skip to the second choice. You may also want to skip to options two or three if you aren't fond of a particular smell and wish to use a different one.

In addition to the three oils recommended to enhance each strength, there is also a counterbalance oil. The counterbalance oil is chosen to give the opposite result. When one strength is overpowering the others and you want it to take the back seat, or when a strength is sabotaging a situation, you may want to tone it down with the counterbalance oil. For example, if you are spending too much time weighing your options, it will help you make a decision. If you are flitting from one task to the next without ever completing a project, the counterbalance oil will help you stay resolute and finish the task.

Example:

Achiever® has three anchor oils. They are Arborvitae, Fennel, and Wild Orange. Arborvitae is the number one choice for Achiever®. However, if you are already using Arborvitae for Deliberative®, you can move on to Fennel. Or if you do not like the smell of Arborvitae, you can choose Fennel or Wild Orange.

The counterbalance oil is Vetiver. Vetiver evokes the opposite of Achiever®. While Achiever® wants to move swiftly forward, Vetiver encourages staying put and being firmly planted in place.

ACHIEVER®

THEME DESCRIPTION

Your Achiever® theme helps explain your drive. Achiever® describes a constant need for achievement. You feel as if every day starts at zero. By the end of the day you must achieve something tangible in order to feel good about yourself. And by "every day" you mean every single day—workdays, weekends, vacations. No matter how much you may feel you deserve a day of rest, if the day passes without some form of achievement, no matter how small, you will feel dissatisfied. You have an internal fire burning inside you. It pushes you to do more, to achieve more. After each accomplishment is reached, the fire dwindles for a moment, but very soon it rekindles itself, forcing you toward the next accomplishment. Your relentless need for achievement might not be logical. It might not even be focused. But it will always be with you. As an Achiever®, you must learn to live with this whisper of discontent. It does have its benefits. It brings you the energy you need to work long hours without burning out. It is the jolt you can always count on to get you started on new tasks, new challenges. It is the power supply that causes you to set the pace and define the levels of productivity for your workgroup. It is the theme that keeps you moving.

ANCHOR OILS

Arborvitae	*Thuja plicata*
Steam-distilled from wood pulp, Arborvitae has a fresh-cut woody smell. It is associated with words such as *composed, driven, long life,* and *power.*	
Fennel	*Foeniculum vulgare*
Fennel, steam-distilled from seeds, is spicy-sweet with a common association of a licorice smell. It is associated with prosperity and flourishing.	
Wild Orange	*Citrus sinensis*
Wild Orange essential oil is cold-pressed from the rind. It is fresh, sweet, and citrusy. Wild Orange inspires abundance. It is encouraging and motivating, and it inspires hard work.	

 COUNTERBALANCE OIL

Vetiver	*Vetiveria zizanioides*
Steam-distilled from the root, Vetiver has a heavy earth smell. It evokes feelings of being deeply grounded and planted.	

ACTIVATOR®

THEME DESCRIPTION

"When can we start?" This is a recurring question in your life. You are impatient for action. You may concede that analysis has its uses or that debate and discussion can occasionally yield some valuable insights, but deep down you know that only action is real. Only action can make things happen. Only action leads to performance. Once a decision is made, you cannot not act. Others may worry that "there are still some things we don't know," but this doesn't seem to slow you. If the decision has been made to go across town, you know that the fastest way to get there is to go stoplight to stoplight. You are not going to sit around waiting until all the lights have turned green. Besides, in your view, action and thinking are not opposites. In fact, guided by your Activator® theme, you believe that action is the best device for learning. You make a decision, you take action, you look at the result, and you learn. This learning informs your next action and your next. How can you grow if you have nothing to react to? Well, you believe you can't. You must put yourself out there. You must take the next step. It is the only way to keep your thinking fresh and informed.

The bottom line is this: You know you will be judged not by what you say, not by what you think, but by what you get done. This does not frighten you. It pleases you.

ANCHOR OILS

Blue Tansy	*Tanacetum annuum*

Blue Tansy is steam-distilled from the flower, leaf, and stem. It has a strong, sweet floral smell. Blue Tansy takes ideas and puts them into action. It spurs the procrastinator toward progress and encourages initiative.

Lemongrass	*Cymbopogon flexuosus*

Lemongrass is steam-distilled from the leaf. It is not a citrus fruit but has a powerful bitter lemon smell, with a hint of earthy grass. Lemongrass is powerful in helping to shed an oil skin and start renewed. It is the antithesis of lethargy.

Eucalyptus	*Eucalyptus radiata*

Eucalyptus is steam-distilled from the leaf and has a sweet, camphor-like smell. It is a very stimulating oil that can foster activity and a healthy perspective.

 COUNTERBALANCE OIL

Vetiver	*Vetiveria zizanioides*

Steam-distilled from the root, Vetiver has a heavy earthy smell. It encourages a feeling of being rooted and still. It calms the mind and supports a firm foundation and blooming where you are planted.

ADAPTABILITY®

THEME DESCRIPTION

You live in the moment. You don't see the future as a fixed destination. Instead, you see it as a place that you create out of the choices that you make right now. And so, you discover your future one choice at a time. This doesn't mean that you don't have plans. You probably do. But this theme of Adaptability® does enable you to respond willingly to the demands of the moment, even if they pull you away from your plans. Unlike some, you don't resent sudden requests or unforeseen detours. You expect them. They are inevitable. Indeed, on some level, you actually look forward to them. You are, at heart, a very flexible person who can stay productive when the demands of work are pulling you in many different directions at once.

ANCHOR OILS

Rosemary	*Rosmarinus officinalis*
Rosemary, steam-distilled from the leaf, has a strong, herbaceous smell. It awakens the mind and keeps one open to new possibilities.	
Cypress	*Cupressus sempervirens*
Cypress, steam-distilled from the leaf, has a fresh, herbaceous aroma with an evergreen undertone. Cypress keeps things moving forward. It is the oil of progression.	
Cilantro	*Coriandrum sativum*
Steam-distilled from the leaf, Cilantro has a fresh, herbaceous aroma with a slight woodsy smell. Cilantro is easygoing. It supports the idea of going with the flow and letting go of the idea that is there only one right way to get something done.	

 COUNTERBALANCE OIL

Neroli	*Citrus aurantium*
Steam-distilled from the flower, Neroli has a light, sweet smell with a deeper bitter second tone. Neroli assists feelings of commitment, especially in partnerships.	

ANALYTICAL®

THEME DESCRIPTION

Your Analytical® theme challenges other people: "Prove it. Show me why what you are claiming is true." In the face of this kind of questioning some will find that their brilliant theories wither and die. For you, this is precisely the point. You do not necessarily want to destroy other people's ideas, but you do insist that their theories be sound. You see yourself as objective and dispassionate. You like data because they are value free. They have no agenda. Armed with these data, you search for patterns and connections. You want to understand how certain patterns affect one another. How do they combine? What is their outcome? Does this outcome fit with the theory being offered or the situation being confronted? These are your questions. You peel the layers back until, gradually, the root cause or causes are revealed.

Others see you as logical and rigorous. Over time they will come to you in order to expose someone's "wishful thinking" or "clumsy thinking" to your refining mind. It is hoped that your analysis is never delivered too harshly. Otherwise, others may avoid you when that "wishful thinking" is their own.

ANCHOR OILS

Geranium	*Pelargonium graveolens*

Steam-distilled from the leaf, Geranium has a green floral scent. Geranium quells distrust and encourages one to look at the situation and have confidence in what one is seeing.

Clove	*Eugenia caryophyllata*

Steam-distilled from the clove bud, Clove has a warm, woodsy, spicy, aroma. Clove instills a belief in self. No need to rely on the opinions of others when you trust your research.

Grapefruit	*Citrus X paradisi*

Cold-pressed from the rind, Grapefruit has a refreshing, citrusy, and bitter smell. It instills self-love through personal validation.

 COUNTERBALANCE OIL

Cilantro	*Coriandrum sativum*

Steam-distilled from the leaf, Cilantro has a fresh, herbaceous aroma, with a slight woodsy smell. Cilantro is easygoing. It supports the idea of going with the flow and letting go of the idea that there is only one right way to get something done.

ARRANGER®

THEME DESCRIPTION

You are a conductor. When faced with a complex situation involving many factors, you enjoy managing all of the variables, aligning and realigning them until you are sure you have arranged them in the most productive configuration possible. In your mind, there is nothing special about what you are doing. You are simply trying to figure out the best way to get things done. But others, lacking this theme, will be in awe of your ability. "How can you keep so many things in your head at once?" They will ask, "How can you stay so flexible, so willing to shelve well-laid plans in favor of some brand-new configuration that has just occurred to you?" But you cannot imagine behaving in any other way. You are a shining example of effective flexibility, whether you are changing travel schedules at the last minute because a better fare has popped up or mulling over just the right combination of people and resources to accomplish a new project. From the mundane to the complex, you are always looking for the perfect configuration.

Of course, you are at your best in dynamic situations. Confronted with the unexpected, some complain that plans devised with such care cannot be changed, while others take refuge in the existing rules or procedures. You don't do either. Instead, you jump into the confusion, devising new options, hunting for new paths of least resistance, and figuring out new partnerships—because, after all, there might just be a better way.

ANCHOR OILS

Douglas Fir	*Pseudotsuga menziesii*

Douglas Fir is steam-distilled from the needles and branches. It has a clean, fresh, pine forest smell. Douglas Fir encourages wisdom to take center stage. With multiple factors coming into play, focus on the obvious truth to solve the problem.

Petitgrain	*Citrus aurantium*

Petitgrain is steam-distilled from the leaf and twigs. It has a complex smell that is floral and woody at the same time. Petitgrain promotes mental clarity.

Lemon	*Citrus limon*

Lemon is cold-pressed from the rind. Lemon has a sharp, bright, and citrusy scent. Lemon supports clarity and focus while casting aside mental confusion and distractibility.

 # COUNTERBALANCE OIL

Tangerine	*Citrus reticulata*

Tangerine is cold-pressed from the rind. It has a sweet citrus smell. If the drive to arrange and fix is being counterproductive, use Tangerine to free you from the responsibility and duty. Tangerine lightens the overburdened mind.

BELIEF®

THEME DESCRIPTION

If you possess a strong Belief® theme, you have certain core values that are enduring. These values vary from one person to another, but ordinarily your Belief® theme causes you to be family oriented, altruistic, even spiritual, and to value responsibility and high ethics—both in yourself and others. These core values affect your behavior in many ways. They give your life meaning and satisfaction; in your view, success is more than money and prestige. They provide you with direction, guiding you through the temptations and distractions of life toward a consistent set of priorities. This consistency is the foundation for all your relationships. Your friends call you dependable. "I know where you stand," they say. Your Belief® makes you easy to trust. It also demands that you find work that meshes with your values. Your work must be meaningful; it must matter to you. And guided by your Belief® theme it will matter only if it gives you a chance to live out your values.

ANCHOR OILS

Roman Chamomile	*Athemis nobilis*

Roman Chamomile is steam-distilled from the flower petals. It has a fruity and floral scent. Roman chamomile drives purpose. It aligns one's actions to one's beliefs.

Sandalwood	*Santalum album*

Sandalwood is steam-distilled from the wood, and as such it has an earthy, woody scent. Sandalwood supports devotion and loyalty.

Spikenard	*Nardostachys jatamansi*

Steam-distilled from the roots, Spikenard has an earthy, musty smell. It is very calming and evokes a feeling of tranquility.

 COUNTERBALANCE OIL

Rosemary	*Rosmarinus officinalis*

Rosemary, steam-distilled from the leaf, has a strong, herbaceous smell. While Belief® often leads one to one sure way of doing things, Rosemary offers new paths and keeps the mind open to new points of view.

COMMAND®

THEME DESCRIPTION

Command® leads you to take charge. Unlike some people, you feel
no discomfort with imposing your views on others. On the contrary,
once your opinion is formed, you need to share it with others. Once
your goal is set, you feel restless until you have aligned others with
you. You are not frightened by confrontation; rather, you know that
confrontation is the first step toward resolution. Whereas others
may avoid facing up to life's unpleasantness, you feel compelled to
present the facts or the truth, no matter how unpleasant it may be.
You need things to be clear between people and challenge them to
be clear-eyed and honest. You push them to take risks. You may
even intimidate them. And while some may resent this, labeling you
opinionated, they often willingly hand you the reins. People are
drawn toward those who take a stance and ask them to move in a
certain direction. Therefore, people will be drawn to you. You have
presence. You have Command®.

ANCHOR OILS

Cassia	*Cinnamomum cassia*
Cassia is steam-distilled from the bark. It has a warm, spicy scent similar to Cinnamon, but sweeter. Cassia is a very bold essential oil that supports self-proclamation.	
Peppermint	*Menta piperita*
Steam-distilled from the leaf, Peppermint has an intense, fresh, mint smell. Peppermint is a dominant oil that is strong and influential. Peppermint is invigorating and takes command.	
Oregano	*Origanum vulgare*
Oregano is steam-distilled from the leaf. It has a strong, herbaceous smell. Oregano is powerful and unyielding.	

 COUNTERBALANCE OIL

Cilantro	*Coriandrum sativum*
Steam-distilled from the leaf, Cilantro is fresh and herbaceous, with a slight woodsy smell. Cilantro is easygoing. It supports the idea of going with the flow, following the crowd, and being a team player.	

COMMUNICATION®

THEME DESCRIPTION

You like to explain, to describe, to host, to speak in public, and to write. This is your Communication® theme at work. Ideas are a dry beginning. Events are static. You feel a need to bring them to life, to energize them, to make them exciting and vivid. And so, you turn events into stories and practice telling them. You take the dry idea and enliven it with images and examples and metaphors. You believe that most people have a very short attention span. They are bombarded by information, but very little of it survives. You want your information—whether an idea, an event, a product's features and benefits, a discovery, or a lesson—to survive. You want to divert their attention toward you and then capture it, lock it in. This is what drives your hunt for the perfect phrase. This is what draws you toward dramatic words and powerful word combinations. This is why people like to listen to you. Your word pictures pique their interest, sharpen their world, and inspire them to action.

ANCHOR OILS

Lavender	*Lavendula angustifolia*

Lavender is steam-distilled from the flower. It has a floral aroma with slight woody undertones. Lavender is the oil of oral expression. It supports honest communication and feeling heard.

Spearmint	*Mentha spicata*

Spearmint is steam-distilled from the whole plant. It has a fresh, light, and minty scent, but the scent is subdued compared to Peppermint. Spearmint is the oil of powerful language. It emboldens one to speak with influence.

Lime	*Citrus aurantifolia*

Lime is cold-pressed from the rind. Lime has a citrusy, sour, and fresh aroma. Use Lime for clearing the air, speaking freely and honestly, and looking forward with brightness.

 COUNTERBALANCE OIL

Cinnamon	*Cinnamomum zeylanicum*

Cinnamon is steam-distilled from the bark. It has a warm, spicy, and earthy smell. Cinnamon allows one to be receptive—to take time to listen rather than speak.

COMPETITION®

THEME DESCRIPTION

Competition® is rooted in comparison. When you look at the world, you are instinctively aware of other people's performance. Their performance is the ultimate yardstick. No matter how hard you tried, no matter how worthy your intentions, if you reached your goal but did not outperform your peers, the achievement feels hollow. Like all competitors, you need other people. You need to compare. If you can compare, you can compete, and if you can compete, you can win. And when you win, there is no feeling quite like it. You like measurement because it facilitates comparisons. You like other competitors because they invigorate you. You like contests because they must produce a winner. You particularly like contests where you know you have the inside track to be the winner. Although you are gracious to your fellow competitors and even stoic in defeat, you don't compete for the fun of competing. You compete to win. Over time you will come to avoid contests where winning seems unlikely.

ANCHOR OILS

Juniper Berry	*Juniperus communis*
Juniper Berry is steam-distilled from the berry. It has a sweet, woody, and zesty aroma. Juniper Berry brings courage and quells fear.	
Cassia	*Cinnamomum cassia*
Cassia is steam-distilled from the bark. It has a warm, spicy scent similar to Cinnamon, but sweeter. Cassia is a very bold essential oil that supports one's own brilliance.	
Siberian Fir	*Abies sibirica*
Steam-distilled from the needles and twigs, Siberian Fir has a fresh pine smell. Siberian Fir boosts the desire to live and leave a legacy. It emboldens and enlivens.	

 COUNTERBALANCE OIL

Thyme	*Thymus vulgaris*
Steam-distilled from the leaf, Thyme has an herbaceous, slightly medicinal, and sweet scent. Thyme is yielding and accepts that while we may not always come in first place, we can always learn from the experience.	

CONNECTEDNESS®

THEME DESCRIPTION

Things happen for a reason. You are sure of it. You are sure of it because in your soul you know that we are all connected. Yes, we are individuals, responsible for our own judgments and in possession of our own free will, but nonetheless we are part of something larger. Some may call it the collective unconscious. Others may label it spirit or life force. But whatever your word of choice, you gain confidence from knowing that we are not isolated from one another or from the earth and the life on it. This feeling of Connectedness® implies certain responsibilities. If we are all part of a larger picture, then we must not harm others because we will be harming ourselves. We must not exploit because we will be exploiting ourselves. Your awareness of these responsibilities creates your value system. You are considerate, caring, and accepting. Certain of the unity of humankind, you are a bridge builder for people of different cultures. Sensitive to the invisible hand, you can give others comfort that there is a purpose beyond our humdrum lives. The exact articles of your faith will depend on your upbringing and your culture, but your faith is strong. It sustains you and your close friends in the face of life's mysteries.

ANCHOR OILS

Cedarwood	*Juniperus virginiana*
Cedarwood, steam-distilled from the bark, has a gentle and woody aroma. Cedarwood instills feelings of community and connection.	
Frankincense	*Boswellia frereana*
Frankincense is steam-distilled from resin. It has a deep, earthy, warm, sweet smell. It is the oil of unification. It connects one to all.	
Marjoram	*Origanum marjorana*
Marjoram is steam-distilled from the leaf. It has a spicy, herbaceous aroma. Marjoram promotes connection in relationships. It bonds.	

 COUNTERBALANCE OIL

Oregano	*Origanum vulgare*
Oregano is steam-distilled from the leaf. It has a strong, herbaceous smell. Oregano is unattached and independent.	

CONSISTENCY®

THEME DESCRIPTION

Balance is important to you. You are keenly aware of the need to treat people the same, no matter what their station in life, so you do not want to see the scales tipped too far in any one person's favor. In your view, this leads to selfishness and individualism. It leads to a world where some people gain an unfair advantage because of their connections or their background or their greasing of the wheels. This is truly offensive to you. You see yourself as a guardian against it. In direct contrast to this world of special favors, you believe that people function best in a consistent environment where the rules are clear and are applied to everyone equally. This is an environment where people know what is expected. It is predictable and evenhanded. It is fair.

Here each person has an even chance to show his or her worth.

ANCHOR OILS

Jasmine	*Jasminum grandiflorum*
Jasmine is an absolute derived from the flowers. It has a deep, honey-like floral smell. Jasmine longs for balance and fairness. It sustains deep intimate relationships based on trust and equity.	
Cedarwood	*Juniperus virginiana*
Cedarwood, steam-distilled from the bark, has a gentle, woody aroma. Cedarwood opens up the mind to connections and supports the collective.	
Patchouli	*Pogostemon cablin*
Patchouli is steam-distilled from the leaf. Patchouli has a slightly sweet and musky aroma. Patchouli encourages balance and alleviates feelings of disconnect.	

 COUNTERBALANCE OIL

Bergamot	*Citrus bergamia*
Bergamot is cold-pressed from the rind. It has a light, fresh, and citrusy aroma. Bergamot recognizes the individual and that not all are the same.	

CONTEXT®

THEME DESCRIPTION

You look back. You look back because that is where the answers lie. You look back to understand the present. From your vantage point, the present is unstable, a confusing clamor of competing voices. It is only by casting your mind back to an earlier time, a time when the plans were being drawn up, that the present regains its stability. The earlier time was a simpler time. It was a time of blueprints. As you look back, you begin to see these blueprints emerge. You realize what the initial intentions were. These blueprints or intentions have since become so embellished that they are almost unrecognizable, but now this Context® theme reveals them again. This understanding brings you confidence. No longer disoriented, you make better decisions because you sense the underlying structure. You become a better partner because you understand how your colleagues came to be who they are.

And counterintuitively you become wiser about the future because you saw its seeds being sown in the past. Faced with new people and new situations, it will take you a little time to orient yourself, but you must give yourself this time. You must discipline yourself to ask the questions and allow the blueprints to emerge because no matter what the situation, if you haven't seen the blueprints, you will have less confidence in your decisions.

ANCHOR OILS

Copaiba	*Copaifera offincinalis*
Steam-distilled from the resin, Copaiba has a mildly sweet, woody smell. Copaiba looks for the connection to the past. By tying the past and present together, copaiba sets the path for a clear and focused future.	

Frankincense	*Boswellia frereana*
Frankincense is steam-distilled from the resin. It has a deep, earthy, warm, sweet smell. It is the oil of unification. It sees the connection between the past, present, and future and the significance of all of them together.	

Siberian Fir	*Abies sibirica*
Steam-distilled from the needles and twigs, Siberian Fir has a fresh pine smell. Looking in the review mirror and connecting generations, Siberian Fir emboldens a desire to live and leave a legacy.	

 COUNTERBALANCE OIL

Clary Sage	*Salvia sclarea*
Clary Sage is steam-distilled from the flower. It has an herbaceous, spicy, and sharp aroma. Clary Sage is considered a visionary oil. It only sees forward. It promotes a clear vision of the path ahead.	

DELIBERATIVE®

THEME DESCRIPTION

You are careful. You are vigilant. You are a private person. You know that the world is an unpredictable place. Everything may seem in order, but beneath the surface you sense the many risks. Rather than denying these risks, you draw each one out into the open. Then each risk can be identified, assessed, and ultimately reduced. Thus, you are a fairly serious person who approaches life with a certain reserve. For example, you like to plan ahead so as to anticipate what might go wrong. You select your friends cautiously and keep your own counsel when the conversation turns to personal matters. You are careful not to give too much praise and recognition, lest it be misconstrued. If some people don't like you because you are not as effusive as others, then so be it. For you, life is not a popularity contest. Life is something of a minefield. Others can run through it recklessly if they so choose, but you take a different approach. You identify the dangers, weigh their relative impact, and then place your feet deliberately. You walk with care.

ANCHOR OILS

Rose	*Rosa damascena*

Steam-distilled from the flowers, Rose has a deep, honey-like floral smell. Rose fosters authenticity and honesty. It is careful with others and promotes awareness through meditation or deep thinking.

Arborvitae	*Thuja plicata*

Steam-distilled from wood pulp, Arborvitae has a fresh-cut woody smell. It is associated with words such as *composed, driven,* and *purposeful.*

Juniper Berry	*Juniperus communis*

Juniper Berry is steam-distilled from the berry. It has a sweet, woody, and zesty aroma. Juniper Berry is insightful and intentional.

 # COUNTERBALANCE OIL

Marjoram	*Origanum marjorana*

Marjoram is steam-distilled from the leaf. It has a spicy, herbaceous smell. Marjoram promotes trust in others and encourages relying on trusted relationships to support the individual.

DEVELOPER®

THEME DESCRIPTION

You see the potential in others. Very often, in fact, potential is all you see. In your view, no individual is fully formed. On the contrary, each individual is a work in progress, alive with possibilities. And you are drawn toward people for this very reason. When you interact with others, your goal is to help them experience success. You look for ways to challenge them. You devise interesting experiences that can stretch them and help them grow. And all the while, you are on the lookout for the signs of growth—a new behavior learned or modified, a slight improvement in a skill, a glimpse of excellence or of "flow" where previously there were only halting steps. For you these small increments—invisible to some—are clear signs of potential being realized. These signs of growth in others are your fuel. They bring you strength and satisfaction. Over time many will seek you out for help and encouragement because on some level they know that your helpfulness is both genuine and fulfilling to you.

ANCHOR OILS

Lemongrass	*Cymbopogon flexuosus*
Lemongrass is steam-distilled from the leaves. It is not a citrus fruit but has a powerful bitter lemon smell with a hint of earthy grass. Lemongrass supports flowing forward, taking something to the next step.	
Myrrh	*Commiphora myrrha*
Myrrh is steam-distilled from the resin. It has an earthy, woody, and balsamic aroma. Myrrh nurtures and develops.	
Patchouli	*Pogostemon cablin*
Patchouli is steam-distilled from the leaf. Patchouli has a slightly sweet and musky aroma. It is an amplifier, enhancing whatever is present.	

 COUNTERBALANCE OIL

Wintergreen	*Gaultheria procumens*
Steam-distilled from the leaves, Wintergreen has a light, fresh, green, and camphor-like smell. Wintergreen helps a stubborn heart let go of needing to be right. It supports acceptance of the way things are without need for change.	

DISCIPLINE®

THEME DESCRIPTION

Your world needs to be predictable. It needs to be ordered and planned. So, you instinctively impose structure on your world. You set up routines. You focus on timelines and deadlines. You break long-term projects into a series of specific short-term plans, and you work through each plan diligently. You are not necessarily neat and clean, but you do need precision. Faced with the inherent messiness of life, you want to feel in control. The routines, the timelines, the structure, all of these helps create this feeling of control. Lacking this theme of Discipline®, others may sometimes resent your need for order, but there need not be conflict. You must understand that not everyone feels your urge for predictability; they have other ways of getting things done. Likewise, you can help them understand and even appreciate your need for structure. Your dislike of surprises, your impatience with errors, your routines, and your detail orientation don't need to be misinterpreted as controlling behaviors that box people in. Rather, these behaviors can be understood as your instinctive method for maintaining your progress and your productivity in the face of life's many distractions.

ANCHOR OILS

Cardamom	*Elettaria cardamomum*
Cardamom is steam-distilled from the seeds. It is sweet and spicy. Cardamom encourages self-control by quelling spontaneity.	
Neroli	*Citrus aurantium*
Neroli is steam-distilled from the flower. It has a sweet floral smell with a slightly bitter afterthought. Neroli promotes commitment, cooperation, and teamwork, especially in partnerships.	
Melaleuca	*Melaleuca alternifolia*
Steam-distilled from the leaf, Melaleuca has an earthy, medicinal scent. It supports a feeling of being collected and whole.	

 COUNTERBALANCE OIL

Petitgrain	*Citrus aurantium*
Petitgrain is steam-distilled from the leaf and twigs. It has a complex smell of being floral and woody at the same time. Petitgrain helps to break habits and break binding chains.	

EMPATHY®

THEME DESCRIPTION

You can sense the emotions of those around you. You can feel what they are feeling as though their feelings are your own. Intuitively, you are able to see the world through their eyes and share their perspective. You do not necessarily agree with each person's perspective. You do not necessarily feel pity for each person's predicament—this would be sympathy, not Empathy®. You do not necessarily condone the choices each person makes, but you do understand. This instinctive ability to understand is powerful. You hear the unvoiced questions. You anticipate the need. Where others grapple for words, you seem to find the right words and the right tone. You help people find the right phrases to express their feelings—to themselves as well as to others. You help them give voice to their emotional life. For all these reasons, other people are drawn to you.

ANCHOR OILS

Myrrh	*Commiphora myrrha*
Myrrh is steam-distilled from the resin. It has an earthy, woody, and balsamic smell. Myrrh promotes nurturing and attachment.	
Lime	*Citrus aurantifolia*
Lime is cold-pressed from the rind. It has a citrusy, sour, and fresh aroma. Lime quells feelings of solitude and detachment and opens the heart.	
Geranium	*Pelargonium graveolens*
Steam-distilled from the leaf, Geranium has a green floral scent. It promotes strong bonds of love and trust.	

 COUNTERBALANCE OIL

Oregano	*Origanum vulgare*
Oregano is steam-distilled from the leaf. It has a strong, herbaceous smell. Oregano is unattached and independent.	

FOCUS®

THEME DESCRIPTION

"Where am I headed?" You ask yourself. You ask this question every day. Guided by this theme of Focus®, you need a clear destination.

Lacking one, your life and your work can quickly become frustrating. And so, each year, each month, and even each week you set goals. These goals then serve as your compass, helping you determine priorities and make the necessary corrections to get back on course. Your Focus® is powerful because it forces you to filter; you instinctively evaluate whether or not a particular action will help you move toward your goal. Those that don't are ignored. In the end, then, your Focus® forces you to be efficient. Naturally, the flip side of this is that it causes you to become impatient with delays, obstacles, and even tangents, no matter how intriguing they appear to be. This makes you an extremely valuable team member. When others start to wander down other avenues, you bring them back to the main road. Your Focus® reminds everyone that if something is not helping you move toward your destination, then it is not important. And if it is not important, then it is not worth your time. You keep everyone on point.

ANCHOR OILS

Vetiver	*Vetiveria zizanioides*
Steam-distilled from the root, Vetiver has a heavy earth smell. It encourages a feeling of being rooted and still. It is very centering.	
Cedarwood	*Juniperus virginiana*
Cedarwood, steam-distilled from the bark, has a gentle, woody aroma. Cedarwood opens up the mind to connections and allows one to be present in the moment by eliminating distractions.	
Lemon	*Citrus limon*
Lemon is cold-pressed from the rind. Lemon has a sharp, bright, and citrusy smell. Lemon supports clarity and focus while casting aside mental confusion and distractibility.	

 COUNTERBALANCE OIL

Rosemary	*Rosmarinus officinalis*
Rosemary, steam-distilled from the leaf, has a strong, herbaceous smell. It awakens the mind and allows it to flow to new ideas and opportunities.	

FUTURISTIC®

THEME DESCRIPTION

"Wouldn't it be great if..." You are the kind of person who loves to peer over the horizon. The future fascinates you. As if it were projected on the wall, you see in detail what the future might hold, and this detailed picture keeps pulling you forward, into tomorrow. While the exact content of the picture will depend on your other strengths and interests—a better product, a better team, a better life, or a better world—it will always be inspirational to you. You are a dreamer who sees visions of what could be and who cherishes those visions. When the present proves too frustrating and the people around you too pragmatic, you conjure up your visions of the future and they energize you. They can energize others, too. In fact, very often people look to you to describe your visions of the future. They want a picture that can raise their sights and thereby their spirits. You can paint it for them. Practice. Choose your words carefully. Make the picture as vivid as possible. People will want to latch on to the hope you bring.

ANCHOR OILS

Clary Sage	*Salvia sclarea*

Clary Sage is steam-distilled from the flower. It has a spicy and sharp, herbaceous aroma. Clary Sage is considered a visionary oil. It promotes a clear vision of your forward path.

Cypress	*Cupressus sempervirens*

Cypress, steam-distilled from the leaf, has a fresh, herbaceous aroma, with an evergreen undertone. Cypress promotes forward thinking. It is the oil of progression.

Geranium	*Pelargonium graveolens*

Steam-distilled from the leaf, Geranium has a green floral scent. It promotes strong bonds of trust that good things are on their way.

 COUNTER BALANCE OIL

Spikenard	*Nardostachys jatamansi*

Steam-distilled from the roots, Spikenard has an earthy, musty smell. Spikenard promotes tranquility and being at peace with the present moment.

HARMONY®

THEME DESCRIPTION

You look for areas of agreement. In your view, there is little to be gained from conflict and friction, so you seek to hold them to a minimum. When you know that the people around you hold differing views, you try to find the common ground. You try to steer them away from confrontation and toward Harmony®. In fact, Harmony® is one of your guiding values. You can't quite believe how much time is wasted by people trying to impose their views on others. Wouldn't we all be more productive if we kept our opinions in check and instead looked for consensus and support? You believe we would, and you live by that belief. When others are sounding off about their goals, their claims, and their fervently held opinions, you hold your peace. When others strike out in a direction, you will willingly, in the service of Harmony®, modify your own objectives to merge with theirs (as long as their basic values do not clash with yours). When others start to argue about their pet theory or concept, you steer clear of the debate, preferring to talk about practical, down-to-earth matters on which you can all agree. In your view, we are all in the same boat, and we need this boat to get where we are going. It is a good boat. There is no need to rock it just to show that you can.

ANCHOR OILS

Petitgrain	*Citrus aurantium*
Petitgrain is steam-distilled from the leaves and twigs. It has a complex smell of being floral and woody at the same time. Petitgrain harmonizes and allows individual parts to work as one.	
Neroli	*Citrus aurantium*
Neroli is steam-distilled from the flower. It has a sweet floral smell with a slightly bitter afterthought. Neroli promotes harmonious partnerships, unification, and teamwork.	
Coriander	*Coriandrum sativum*
Steam-distilled from the seeds, Coriander has a woody, spicy, and sweet aroma. Coriander serves others, even to the point of self-neglect. It is loyal and bonded.	

 COUNTERBALANCE OIL

Cassia	*Cinnamomum cassia*
Cassia is steam-distilled from the bark. It has a warm, spicy scent similar to Cinnamon, but sweeter. Cassia is a very bold essential oil that supports one's own brilliance. It is unashamed.	

IDEATION®

THEME DESCRIPTION

You are fascinated by ideas. What is an idea? An idea is a concept,
the best explanation of the most events. You are delighted when you
discover beneath the complex surface an elegantly simple concept
to explain why things are the way they are. An idea is a connection.
Yours is the kind of mind that is always looking for connections,
and so you are intrigued when seemingly disparate phenomena can
be linked by an obscure connection. An idea is a new perspective on
familiar challenges. You revel in taking the world we all know and
turning it around so we can view it from a strange but strangely
enlightening angle. You love all these ideas because they are
profound, because they are novel, because they are clarifying,
because they are contrary, because they are bizarre. For all these
reasons, you derive a jolt of energy whenever a new idea occurs to
you. Others may label you creative or original or conceptual or
even smart. Perhaps you are all of these. Who can be sure? What
you are sure of is that ideas are thrilling. And on most days, this is
enough.

ANCHOR OILS

Tangerine	*Citrus reticulata*

Cold-pressed from the rind, Tangerine has a bright, fresh, and citrusy aroma. Tangerine is uplifting and encourages creativity, allowing for new and fresh ideas to spring forth.

Clary Sage	*Salvia sclarea*

Clary Sage is steam-distilled from the flower. It has a spicy, sharp, and herbaceous aroma. Clary Sage is considered a visionary oil. It promotes a clear vision, clarity, and an enlightened path.

Juniper Berry	*Juniperus communis*

Juniper Berry is steam-distilled from the berry. It has sweet, woody, and zesty scent. Juniper Berry releases tension and "feeling stuck." It promotes insight and ideas.

 COUNTERBALANCE OIL

Vetiver	*Vetiveria zizanioides*

Steam-distilled from the root, Vetiver has a heavy earth smell. It encourages a feeling of being rooted and still. It calms the mind and brings it to a central focus.

INCLUDER®

THEME DESCRIPTION

"Stretch the circle wider." This is the philosophy around which you orient your life. You want to include people and make them feel part of the group. In direct contrast to those who are drawn only to exclusive groups, you actively avoid those groups that exclude others. You want to expand the group so that as many people as possible can benefit from its support. You hate the sight of someone on the outside looking in. You want to draw them in so that they can feel the warmth of the group. You are an instinctively accepting person.

Regardless of race or sex or nationality or personality or faith, you cast few judgments. Judgments can hurt a person's feelings. Why do that if you don't have to? Your accepting nature does not necessarily rest on a belief that each of us is different and that one should respect these differences. Rather, it rests on your conviction that fundamentally we are all the same. We are all equally important. Thus, no one should be ignored. Each of us should be included. It is the least we all deserve.

ANCHOR OILS

Melaleuca	*Melaleuca alternifolia*

Melaleuca is steam-distilled from the leaf. It has an earthy, medicinal scent. Melaleuca helps with feeling collected and whole.

Cedarwood	*Juniperus virginiana*

Cedarwood, steam-distilled from the bark, has a gentle and woody aroma. Cedarwood promotes the belief that there is strength in the collective. It supports community.

Frankincense	*Boswellia frereana*

Frankincense is steam-distilled from resin. It has a deep, earthy, warm, sweet smell. It is the oil of unification. It sees the connection between the past, present, and future, and the significance of all of them together.

 # COUNTERBALANCE OIL

Clove	*Eugenia caryophyllata*

Steam-distilled from the clove bud, Clove has a warm, woodsy, spicy, aroma. Clove instills a belief in self. No need to rely on the opinions of others when you trust yourself. Clove supports healthy boundaries.

INDIVIDUALIZATION®

THEME DESCRIPTION

Your Individualization® theme leads you to be intrigued by the unique qualities of each person. You are impatient with generalizations or "types" because you don't want to obscure what is special and distinct about each person. Instead, you focus on the differences between individuals. You instinctively observe each person's style, each person's motivation, how each thinks, and how each builds relationships. You hear the one-of-a-kind stories in each person's life. This theme explains why you pick your friends just the right birthday gift, why you know that one person prefers praise in public and another detests it, and why you tailor your teaching style to accommodate one person's need to be shown and another's desire to "figure it out as I go." Because you are such a keen observer of other people's strengths, you can draw out the best in each person. This Individualization® theme also helps you build productive teams. While some search around for the perfect team "structure" or "process," you know instinctively that the secret to great teams is casting by individual strengths so that everyone can do a lot of what they do well.

ANCHOR OILS

Black Pepper	*Piper nigrum*

Black Pepper is steam-distilled from the berry. It has a dark, spicy, and peppery smell. Black Pepper encourages the shedding of the facade and revealing the true individual self.

Bergamot	*Citrus bergamia*

Bergamot is cold-pressed from the rind. It has a light, fresh, and citrusy aroma. Bergamot recognizes the individual and that there is power and strength in standing on your own.

Coriander	*Coriandrum sativum*

Steam-distilled from the seeds, Coriander has a woody, spicy, and sweet scent. Coriander sees each person as a gift. It allows one to view others as unique and special.

 COUNTERBALANCE OIL

Cedarwood	*Juniperus virginiana*

Cedarwood, steam-distilled from the bark, has a gentle and woody aroma. Cedarwood opens the mind to connections and sees how each individual plays a part in the bigger picture.

INPUT®

THEME DESCRIPTION

You are inquisitive. You collect things. You might collect information—words, facts, books, and quotations—or you might collect tangible objects such as butterflies, baseball cards, porcelain dolls, or sepia photographs. Whatever you collect, you collect it because it interests you. And yours is the kind of mind that finds so many things interesting. The world is exciting precisely because of its infinite variety and complexity. If you read a great deal, it is not necessarily to refine your theories but, rather, to add more information to your archives. If you like to travel, it is because each new location offers novel artifacts and facts. These can be acquired and then stored away. Why are they worth storing? At the time of storing it is often hard to say exactly when or why you might need them, but who knows when they might become useful? With all those possible uses in mind, you really don't feel comfortable throwing anything away. So, you keep acquiring and compiling and filing stuff away. It's interesting. It keeps your mind fresh. And perhaps one day some of it will prove valuable.

ANCHOR OILS

Siberian Fir	*Abies sibirica*

Steam-distilled from the needles and twigs, Siberian Fir has a fresh pine smell. Siberian Fir is an oil of assessment and reflection. It supports the collection of thoughts and stories in order to make empowered decisions.

Lavender	*Lavendula angustifolia*

Lavender is steam-distilled from the flower. It has a floral scent with slight woody undertones. Lavender is an oil that supports expression. When you've gathered all the needed information, Lavender will help you share the data in a meaningful way.

Rosemary	*Rosmarinus officinalis*

Rosemary, steam-distilled from the leaf, has a strong, herbaceous smell. Rosemary is a powerful essential oil associated with the mind and memory recall. Learning new information is great, but remembering it when you need it is just as valuable.

 COUNTERBALANCE OIL

Clove	*Eugenia caryophyllata*

Steam-distilled from the clove bud, Clove has a warm, woodsy, spicy aroma. Clove supports healthy boundaries. It's important to know when you have enough and to move out of the research stage and take action.

INTELLECTION®

THEME DESCRIPTION

You like to think. You like mental activity. You like exercising the "muscles" of your brain, stretching them in multiple directions. This need for mental activity may be focused; for example, you may be trying to solve a problem or develop an idea or understand another person's feelings. The exact focus will depend on your other strengths. On the other hand, this mental activity may very well lack focus. The theme of Intellection® does not dictate what you are thinking about; it simply describes that you like to think. You are the kind of person who enjoys your time alone because it is your time for musing and reflection. You are introspective. In a sense, you are your own best companion, as you pose yourself questions and try out answers on yourself to see how they sound. This introspection may lead you to a slight sense of discontent as you compare what you are actually doing with all the thoughts and ideas that your mind conceives. Or this introspection may tend toward more pragmatic matters such as the events of the day or a conversation that you plan to have later. Wherever it leads you, this mental hum is one of the constants of your life.

ANCHOR OILS

Frankincense	*Boswellia frereana*

Frankincense is steam-distilled from resin. It has a deep, earthy, warm, sweet smell. Frankincense supports truth. It enlivens the mind to knowledge and learning.

Rosemary	*Rosmarinus officinalis*

Rosemary, steam-distilled from the leaf, has a strong, herbaceous smell. Rosemary is a powerful essential oil associated with the mind and memory. It is the oil of the mind.

Siberian Fir	*Abies sibirica*

Steam-distilled from the needles and twigs, Siberian Fir has a fresh pine smell. Siberian Fir is an oil of assessment and reflection. It supports the collection of thoughts and stories in order to make empowered decisions.

 COUNTERBALANCE OIL

Spearmint	*Mentha spicata*

Spearmint is steam-distilled from the whole plant. It has a fresh, light, and minty aroma, but it is subdued compared to Peppermint. Spearmint is the oil of powerful language. It emboldens one to get out of one's head and speak one's mind.

LEARNER®

THEME DESCRIPTION

You love to learn. The subject matter that interests you most will be determined by your other themes and experiences, but whatever the subject, you will always be drawn to the process of learning. The process, more than the content or the result, is especially exciting for you. You are energized by the steady and deliberate journey from ignorance to competence. The thrill of the first few facts, the early efforts to recite or practice what you have learned, the growing confidence of a skill mastered—this is the process that entices you. Your excitement leads you to engage in adult learning experiences—yoga or piano lessons or graduate classes. It enables you to thrive in dynamic work environments where you are asked to take on short project assignments and are expected to learn a lot about the new subject matter in a short period of time and then move on to the next one. This Learner® theme does not necessarily mean that you seek to become the subject matter expert or that you are striving for the respect that accompanies a professional or academic credential. The outcome of the learning is less significant than the "getting there."

ANCHOR OILS

Melissa	*Melissa officinalis*

Steam-distilled from the leaf and flower, Melissa is a precious oil with a delicate and spicy flower scent. It supports elevating to higher realms of enlightenment.

Rosemary	*Rosmarinus officinalis*

Rosemary, steam-distilled from the leaf, has a strong, herbaceous smell. Rosemary is a powerful essential oil associated with the mind and memory. It is the oil of the mind.

Douglas Fir	*Pseudotsuga menziesii*

Douglas Fir is steam-distilled from the needles and branches. It has a clean, fresh, pine forest smell. Douglas Fir encourages wisdom to take center stage.

 COUNTERBALANCE OIL

Ginger	*Zingiber officinale*

Often described as spicy, woody, fresh, and sharp, Ginger is steam-distilled from the root. It is an empowering oil that encourages action. You have learned enough. Now it is time to act on that knowledge.

MAXIMIZER®

THEME DESCRIPTION

Excellence, not average, is your measure. Taking something from
below average to slightly above average takes a great deal of effort
and in your opinion, is not very rewarding. Transforming something
strong into something superb takes just as much effort but is much
more thrilling. Strengths, whether yours or someone else's, fascinate
you. Like a diver after pearls, you search them out, watching for the
telltale signs of a strength. A glimpse of untutored excellence, rapid
learning, a skill mastered without recourse to steps—all these are
clues that a strength may be in play. And having found a strength, you
feel compelled to nurture it, refine it, and stretch it toward excellence.
You polish the pearl until it shines. This natural sorting of strengths
means that others see you as discriminating. You choose to spend
time with people who appreciate your particular strengths. Likewise,
you are attracted to others who seem to have found and cultivated
their own strengths. You tend to avoid those who want to fix you and
make you well rounded. You don't want to spend your life bemoaning
what you lack. Rather, you want to capitalize on the gifts with which
you are blessed. It's more fun. It's more productive. And,
counterintuitively, it is more demanding.

ANCHOR OILS

Patchouli	*Pogostemon cablin*
Patchouli is steam-distilled from the leaf. Patchouli has a slightly sweet and musky aroma. Patchouli supports taking it to the next level. It maximizes opportunities and potential.	
Copaiba	*Copaifera offincinalis*
Steam-distilled from the resin, Copaiba has a mildly sweet, woody smell. Copaiba maximizes potential and galvanizes purposeful living.	
Fennel	*Foeniculum vulgare*
Steam-distilled from the seeds, Fennel has a licorice-like smell that is spicy and sweet. Fennel supports flourishing and blooming where you are planted.	

 ## COUNTERBALANCE OIL

Bergamot	*Citrus bergamia*
Bergamot is cold-pressed from the rind. It has a light, fresh, and citrusy aroma. Bergamot supports self-acceptance, supporting that you are valuable just the way you are with no need to prove yourself or change yourself to please others.	

POSITIVITY®

THEME DESCRIPTION

You are generous with praise, quick to smile, and always on the lookout for the positive in the situation. Some call you lighthearted. Others just wish that their glass were as full as yours seems to be. But either way, people want to be around you. Their world looks better around you because your enthusiasm is contagious. Lacking your energy and optimism, some find their world drab with repetition or, worse, heavy with pressure. You seem to find a way to lighten their spirit. You inject drama into every project. You celebrate every achievement. You find ways to make everything more exciting and more vital. Some cynics may reject your energy, but you are rarely dragged down. Your Positivity® won't allow it. Somehow you can't quite escape your conviction that it is good to be alive, that work can be fun, and that no matter what the setbacks, one must never lose one's sense of humor.

ANCHOR OILS

Ylang Ylang	*Cananga odorata*
Steam-distilled from the flower, Ylang Ylang has a very heavy sweetness, reminiscent of a tropical floral scent. Ylang Ylang is an oil that personifies exuberant joy.	
Tangerine	*Citrus reticulata*
Cold-pressed from the rind, Tangerine has a bright, fresh, and citrusy aroma. Tangerine is uplifting and encourages creativity, allowing for new and fresh ideas to spring forth.	
Lime	*Citrus aurantifolia*
Lime is cold-pressed from the rind. It has a citrusy, sour, and fresh scent. Lime opens the heart and increases zest for life.	

 COUNTERBALANCE OIL

Black Pepper	*Piper nigrum*
Black Pepper is steam-distilled from the berry. It has a dark spicy peppery smell. Black Pepper encourages acceptance of things the way they are. It is based in reality and allows for honest evaluation and removal of the rose-colored glasses.	

RELATOR®

THEME DESCRIPTION

Relator® describes your attitude toward your relationships. In simple terms, the Relator® theme pulls you toward people you already know. You do not necessarily shy away from meeting new people—in fact, you may have other themes that cause you to enjoy the thrill of turning strangers into friends—but you do derive a great deal of pleasure and strength from being around your close friends. You are comfortable with intimacy. Once the initial connection has been made, you deliberately encourage a deepening of the relationship.

You want to understand their feelings, their goals, their fears, and their dreams; and you want them to understand yours. You know that this kind of closeness implies a certain amount of risk—you might be taken advantage of—but you are willing to accept that risk. For you a relationship has value only if it is genuine. And the only way to know that is to entrust yourself to the other person. The more you share with each other, the more you risk together. The more you risk together, the more each of you proves your caring is genuine. These are your steps toward real friendship, and you take them willingly.

ANCHOR OILS

Marjoram	*Origanum majorana*

Steam-distilled from the leaf, Marjoram has a spicy, herbaceous aroma. It is the oil of trust. It supports deep meaningful relationships.

Cedarwood	*Juniperus virginiana*

Cedarwood, steam-distilled from the bark, has a gentle and woody aroma. Cedarwood promotes the belief that there is strength in the collective. It supports community.

Coriander	*Coriandrum sativum*

Steam-distilled from the seeds, Coriander has a woody, spicy, and sweet scent. Coriander honors integrity, which is so important to a Relator®.

 COUNTERBALANCE OIL

Rosemary	*Rosmarinus officinalis*

Rosemary, steam-distilled from the leaf, has a strong, herbaceous smell. Rosemary is a powerful essential oil associated with the mind and memory. It is the oil of the mind.

RESPONSIBILITY®

THEME DESCRIPTION

Your Responsibility® theme forces you to take psychological
ownership for anything you commit to, and whether large or small,
you feel emotionally bound to follow it through to completion. Your
good name depends on it. If for some reason you cannot deliver, you
automatically start to look for ways to make it up to the other person.
Apologies are not enough. Excuses and rationalizations are totally
unacceptable. You will not quite be able to live with yourself until you
have made restitution. This conscientiousness, this near obsession for
doing things right, and your impeccable ethics, combine to create your
reputation: utterly dependable. When assigning new responsibilities,
people will look to you first because they know it will get done. When
people come to you for help—and they soon will—you must be
selective. Your willingness to volunteer may sometimes lead you to
take on more than you should.

ANCHOR OILS

Fennel	*Foeniculum vulgare*
Steam-distilled from the seeds, Fennel has a licorice-like smell that is spicy and sweet. Fennel supports taking responsibility for where you are. Take ownership of your destiny and your life situation.	
Ginger	*Zingiber officinale*
Often described as spicy, woody, fresh, and sharp, Ginger is steam-distilled from the root. It is an empowering oil that encourages action. You are responsible for your knowledge and gifts—now act on them.	
Cardamom	*Elettaria cardamomum*
Cardamom is steam-distilled from the seeds. It has a sweet and spicy aroma. Cardamom encourages self-control, integrity, and levelheadedness.	

 COUNTERBALANCE OIL

Ylang Ylang	*Cananga odorata*
Steam-distilled from the flower, Ylang Ylang has a very heavy sweetness, reminiscent of a tropical floral scent. Ylang Ylang is an oil that personifies exuberant joy. It unleashes the inner child and allows one to enjoy the moment instead of feeling the weight of the world on one's shoulders.	

RESTORATIVE™

THEME DESCRIPTION

You love to solve problems. Whereas some are dismayed when they encounter yet another breakdown, you can be energized by it. You enjoy the challenge of analyzing the symptoms, identifying what is wrong, and finding the solution. You may prefer practical problems or conceptual ones or personal ones. You may seek out specific kinds of problems that you have met many times before and that you are confident you can fix. Or you may feel the greatest push when faced with complex and unfamiliar problems. Your exact preferences are determined by your other themes and experiences. But what is certain is that you enjoy bringing things back to life. It is a wonderful feeling to identify the undermining factor(s), eradicate them, and restore something to its true glory. Intuitively, you know that without your intervention, this thing—this machine, this technique, this person, this company—might have ceased to function. You fixed it, resuscitated it, rekindled its vitality. Phrasing it the way you might, you saved it.

ANCHOR OILS

Basil	*Ocimum basilcum*
Basil is steam-distilled from the leaf. It has a spicy and bright herbaceous aroma. Basil is like a phoenix. It supports arising from the ashes and renewing and restoration. It combats burnout.	
Geranium	*Pelargonium graveolens*
Steam-distilled from the leaf, Geranium has a green floral scent. Geranium promotes mending bonds, mending relationships, and restoring trust.	
Ylang Ylang	*Cananga odorata*
Steam-distilled from the flower, Ylang Ylang has a very heavy sweetness, reminiscent of a tropical floral scent. Ylang Ylang restores one to one's childlike state. It supports joy and simplicity.	

 COUNTER BALANCE OIL

Thyme	*Thymus vulgaris*
Steam-distilled from the leaf, Thyme has a slightly medicinal and sweet, herbaceous smell. Thyme is yielding and accepts that some things are broken, and it is time to move on. It encourages acceptance and forgiveness.	

SELF-ASSURANCE®

THEME DESCRIPTION

Self-Assurance® is similar to self-confidence. In the deepest part of
you, you have faith in your strengths. You know that you are able—
able to take risks, able to meet new challenges, able to stake claims,
and, most important, able to deliver. But Self-Assurance® is more
than just self-confidence. Blessed with the theme of Self-Assurance®,
you have confidence not only in your abilities but in your judgment.
When you look at the world, you know that your perspective is
unique and distinct. And because no one sees exactly what you see,
you know that no one can make your decisions for you. No one can
tell you what to think. They can guide. They can suggest. But you
alone have the authority to form conclusions, make decisions, and
act. This authority, this final accountability for the living of your life,
does not intimidate you. On the contrary, it feels natural to you. No
matter what the situation, you seem to know what the right decision
is. This theme lends you an aura of certainty. Unlike many, you are
not easily swayed by someone else's arguments, no matter how
persuasive they may be. This Self-Assurance® may be quiet or loud,
depending on your other themes, but it is solid. It is strong. Like the
keel of a ship, it withstands many different pressures and keeps you
on your course.

ANCHOR OILS

Bergamot	*Citrus bergamia*

Bergamot is cold-pressed from the rind. It has a light, fresh, and citrusy aroma. Bergamot supports the individual. It encourages self-acceptance and understanding the significance of each person and his or her contribution to the world.

Grapefruit	*Citrus X paradisi*

Cold-pressed from the rind, grapefruit has a refreshing, citrusy, and bitter scent. Grapefruit instills self-love through personal validation.

Ginger	*Zingiber officinale*

Often described as spicy, woody, fresh, and sharp, Ginger is steam-distilled from the root. Ginger is a warrior oil. It is an empowering oil that encourages action. You are responsible for your knowledge and gifts, and you have a personal responsibility to use those gifts and knowledge to have an impact on the world.

 COUNTERBALANCE OIL

Wintergreen	*Gaultheria procumens*

Steam-distilled from the leaves, Wintergreen has a light, fresh, green, and camphor-like aroma. Wintergreen helps a stubborn heart let go of needing to be right. It supports acceptance and surrender.

SIGNIFICANCE®

THEME DESCRIPTION

You want to be very significant in the eyes of other people. In the truest sense of the word you want to be recognized. You want to be heard. You want to stand out. You want to be known. In particular, you want to be known and appreciated for the unique strengths you bring. You feel a need to be admired as credible, professional, and successful. Likewise, you want to associate with others who are credible, professional, and successful. And if they aren't, you will push them to achieve until they are. Or you will move on. An independent spirit, you want your work to be a way of life rather than a job, and in that work, you want to be given free rein, the leeway to do things your way. Your yearnings feel intense to you, and you honor those yearnings. And so, your life is filled with goals, achievements, or qualifications that you crave. Whatever your focus—and each person is distinct—your Significance® theme will keep pulling you upward, away from the mediocre toward the exceptional. It is the theme that keeps you reaching.

ANCHOR OILS

Cinnamon	*Cinnamomum zeylanicum*
Cinnamon is steam-distilled from the bark. It has a warm, spicy, and earthy aroma. Cinnamon allows one to step into one's power. It is an oil that minimizes insecurities, thus allowing empowering vulnerability.	
Spearmint	*Mentha spicata*
Spearmint is steam-distilled from the whole plant. It has a fresh, light, and minty smell, but it is subdued compared to Peppermint. Spearmint is the oil of powerful language. It emboldens one to get out of one's head and speak one's mind. It supports self-worth and holding one's ground.	
Frankincense	*Boswellia frereana*
Frankincense is steam-distilled from resin. It has a deep, earthy, warm, sweet smell. Frankincense supports divine worth. It is known as the king of the oils.	

 COUNTERBALANCE OIL

Oregano	*Origanum vulgare*
Oregano is steam-distilled from the leaf. It has a strong, herbaceous smell. Oregano supports humility.	

STRATEGIC®

THEME DESCRIPTION

The Strategic® theme enables you to sort through the clutter and find the best route. It is not a skill that can be taught. It is a distinct way of thinking, a special perspective on the world at large. This perspective allows you to see patterns where others simply see complexity. Mindful of these patterns, you play out alternative scenarios, always asking, "What if this happened? Okay, well what if this happened?" This recurring question helps you see around the next corner. There you can evaluate accurately the potential obstacles. Guided by where you see each path leading, you start to make selections. You discard the paths that lead nowhere. You discard the paths that lead straight into resistance. You discard the paths that lead into a fog of confusion. You cull and make selections until you arrive at the chosen path—your strategy. Armed with your strategy, you strike forward. This is your Strategic® theme at work: "What if?" Select. Strike.

ANCHOR OILS

Clary Sage	*Salvia sclarea*
Clary Sage is steam-distilled from the flower. It has a spicy, sharp, and herbaceous smell. Clary Sage is considered a visionary oil. It promotes a clear vision of your forward path. It supports following your intuition.	
Vetiver	*Vetiveria zizanioides*
Steam-distilled from the root, Vetiver has a heavy earth smell. It encourages focus around distractions. It can help to center and root among chaos.	
Juniper Berry	*Juniperus communis*
Juniper Berry is steam-distilled from the berry. It has a sweet, woody, and zesty aroma. Juniper Berry releases tension and "feeling stuck." It promotes insight and ideas.	

 COUNTERBALANCE OIL

Lemongrass	*Cymbopogon flexuosus*
Lemongrass is steam-distilled from the leaves. It is not a citrus fruit, but it has a powerful bitter lemon smell with a hint of earthy grass. Lemongrass supports flowing forward, sometimes without direction. It does not need a deliberate path. It is more free-flowing.	

WOO®

THEME DESCRIPTION

Woo® stands for winning others over. You enjoy the challenge of meeting new people and getting them to like you. Strangers are rarely intimidating to you. On the contrary, strangers can be energizing. You are drawn to them. You want to learn their names, ask them questions, and find some area of common interest so that you can strike up a conversation and build rapport. Some people shy away from starting up conversations because they worry about running out of things to say. You don't. Not only are you rarely at a loss for words; you actually enjoy initiating with strangers because you derive satisfaction from breaking the ice and making a connection. Once that connection is made, you are quite happy to wrap it up and move on. There are new people to meet, new rooms to work, new crowds to mingle in. In your world there are no strangers, only friends you haven't met yet—lots of them.

ANCHOR OILS

Ylang Ylang	*Cananga odorata*

Steam-distilled from the flower, Ylang Ylang has a very heavy sweetness, reminiscent of a tropical floral scent. Ylang Ylang is exuberant and joyful. It is playful and interactive.

Jasmine	*Jasminum grandiflorum*

Jasmine is an absolute derived from the flowers. It has a deep, honey-like floral smell. Jasmine desires liberation. By encouraging trust and intimacy quickly, Jasmine supports the development of strong and powerful relationships.

Spearmint	*Mentha spicata*

Spearmint is steam-distilled from the whole plant. It has a fresh, light, and minty aroma, but it is subdued compared to Peppermint. Spearmint is the oil of powerful language. It emboldens, instilling confidence and speed.

 # COUNTERBALANCE OIL

Grapefruit	*Citrus X paradisi*

Cold-pressed from the rind, Grapefruit has a refreshing, citrusy, and bitter aroma. Grapefruit instills self-love through personal validation. Grapefruit helps to break the reliance on other's opinions or approval.

CHAPTER SEVEN:
BLENDING
ESSENTIAL OILS

Blending essential oils is the process of combining several oils with a carrier oil to have a ready-made blend. Using several essential oils together may be necessary to reach a desired outcome. When there are multiple layers to an issue, multiple essential oils may be required to get to the root of the problem. Blending several essential oils together and applying to the skin makes the process easy. And the easier it is, the more likely you are to incorporate it into your daily life. These recipes are pairings or blends of several strengths. While you will not want to anchor a blend to multiple strengths, these blends may help you to "get into the zone" and support mood and mind throughout the day. You can keep your oils on a keychain or in a pouch, or you may want to create an oils station in your bedroom or kitchen. The key is to have them accessible and ready to use.

Apply the essential oil blend to the bottom of the feet to start the day. Use on the wrists or back of the neck throughout the day as needed.

You may also choose to apply your oils to aromatherapy jewelry or as perfume.

To make your own blends, add no more than twenty drops of essential oils per ten-milliliter blend. The remainder of the bottle will be filled with your carrier oil.

Oil blends containing citrus oils can be sun sensitive. Apply these to the bottom of the feet or where they will be covered by clothing. Avoid direct sunlight to the application area for twelve hours.

SUPPLIES NEEDED

Essential oils

Carrier oil (for dilution)

Glass roller bottles (my preference is any dark-colored ten-milliliter glass bottle; these will come with the roller top and cap included)

Labels (make them yourself or buy premade)

If you have an essential oils supplier or educator, I encourage you to go back to them for your purchasing needs.
If not, all supplies, including essential oils, can be purchased from **www.anchortoyourstrengths.com**

DIRECTIONS

Drop the designated essential oils into a glass roller bottle.

Top off the remainder of the roller bottle with a carrier oil. My favorite is fractionated coconut oil. You can also use almond oil, olive oil, jojoba oil, grape-seed oil, and so forth.

Label your bottle.

Roll on your skin or apply to aromatherapy jewelry to tap into your strengths.

The number of drops is indicated in each recipe.

RECITES

■ ■ ■

START TO FINISH

Activator® + Achiever®
♦♦♦♦♦ five drops Lemongrass
♦♦♦ three drops Arborvitae

GO WITH THE FLOW

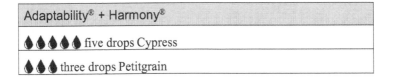

Adaptability® + Harmony®
♦♦♦♦♦ five drops Cypress
♦♦♦ three drops Petitgrain

SEE THE BEST

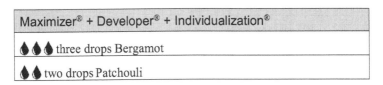

Maximizer® + Developer® + Individualization®
♦♦♦ three drops Bergamot
♦♦ two drops Patchouli

BREAKTHROUGH

Activator® + Command® + Woo®
🔹🔹🔹🔹🔹 five drops Wild Orange
🔹🔹🔹 three drops Ylang Ylang

WINNER'S CIRCLE

Competition® + Harmony® + Woo®
🔹🔹🔹🔹 four drops Spearmint
🔹 one drop Cassia
🔹 one drop Neroli

TRUTH TELLER

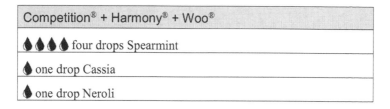

Belief® + Command® + Analytical®
🔹🔹🔹🔹🔹 five drops Roman Chamomile
🔹🔹 two drops Geranium

SOCIAL SPEED

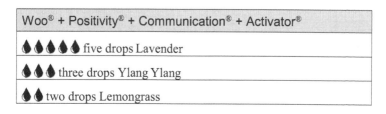

Woo® + Positivity® + Communication® + Activator®
🔹🔹🔹🔹🔹 five drops Lavender
🔹🔹🔹 three drops Ylang Ylang
🔹🔹 two drops Lemongrass

LET ME THINK

Deliberative® + Input® + Intellection®
🌢🌢🌢🌢 four drops Lavender
🌢🌢 two drops Arborvitae
🌢 one drop Rosemary

AUTHENTICITY

Relator® + Responsibility®
🌢🌢🌢🌢 four drops Cardamom
🌢🌢🌢 three drops Cedarwood

ON THE MOVE

Self-Assurance® + Activator® + Strategic® + Achiever®
🌢🌢🌢🌢 four drops Bergamot
🌢🌢 two drops Lemongrass
🌢🌢 two drops Vetiver

IN THE ZONE

Focus® + Intellection® + Self-Assurance®
🌢🌢🌢🌢 four drops Frankincense
🌢🌢🌢🌢 four drops Lemon
🌢🌢 two drops Vetiver

FEELIN' IT

Empathy® + Positivity® + Includer®
⬤⬤⬤⬤ four drops Frankincense
⬤⬤⬤ three drops Lime

TRANSFORMATION

Developer® + Maximizer® + Individualization® + Restorative™
⬤⬤⬤ three drops Ylang Ylang
⬤⬤⬤ three drops Patchouli
⬤⬤ two drops Bergamot

GIVE ME OPTIONS

Ideation® + Strategic® + Futuristic® + Maximizer®
⬤⬤⬤⬤ four drops Tangerine
⬤⬤⬤ three drops Clary Sage
⬤ one drop Basil

TAKE IT SLOW

Deliberative® + Restorative™ + Input® + Intellection®
⬤⬤⬤ three drops Ylang Ylang
⬤⬤⬤ three drops Lavender
⬤⬤ two drops Copaiba

PRESENT

Adaptability® + Focus® + Self-Assurance® + Connectedness® + Empathy®
◆◆◆◆ four drops Frankincense
◆◆ two drops Lime
◆◆ two drops Lemon
◆◆ two drops Grapefruit

FUTURE TENSE

Futuristic® + Belief®
◆◆◆◆ four drops Roman Chamomile
◆◆ two drops Cypress

LOVE ME

Woo® + Significance® + Self-Assurance® + Positivity®
◆◆◆◆◆ five drops Spearmint
◆◆ two drops Grapefruit
◆◆ two drops Lime

PARTNERS

Adaptability® + Developer® + Empathy® + Connectedness®
◆◆◆◆ four drops Myrrh
◆◆◆ three drops Lime

MULTITASKER

Arranger® + Ideation® + Strategic® + Harmony®
◆◆◆ three drops Lemon
◆◆◆ three drops Tangerine
◆ one drop Juniper Berry

LAYING DOWN THE LAW

Discipline® + Consistency® + Command® + Self-Assurance®
◆◆◆◆ four drops Bergamot
◆◆ two drops Cardamom
◆◆ two drops Cedarwood

STORYTELLER

Communication® + Context® + Woo® + Belief®
◆◆◆◆◆ five drops Lavender
◆◆ two drops Frankincense
◆◆ two drops Sandalwood

BEST FRIEND FOREVER

Relator® + Empathy® + Positivity® + Connectedness®
🌢🌢🌢🌢 four drops Lime
🌢🌢 two drops Cedarwood
🌢🌢 two drops Frankincense

103

NOTES

▪ ▪ ▪

MY TOP FIVE

1.

2.

3.

4.

5.

STRENGTH 1

Anchor Oil:

Counterbalance Oil:

Comments:

STRENGTH 2

Anchor Oil:

Counterbalance Oil:

Comments:

STRENGTH 3

Anchor Oil:

Counterbalance Oil:

Comments:

STRENGTH 4

Anchor Oil:

Counterbalance Oil:

Comments:

STRENGTH 5

Anchor Oil:

Counterbalance Oil:

Comments:

NOTES

NOTES

NOTES

APPENDIX:
QUICK REFERENCE GUIDE

Talent Theme	Oil 1	Oil 2	Oil 3	Counterbalance
ACHIEVER®	Arborvitae	Fennel	Wild Orange	Vetiver
ACTIVATOR®	Blue Tansy	Lemongrass	Eucalyptus	Vetiver
ADAPTABILITY®	Rosemary	Cypress	Cilantro	Neroli
ANALYTICAL®	Geranium	Clove	Grapefruit	Cilantro
ARRANGER®	Douglas Fir	Petitgrain	Lemon	Tangerine
BELIEF®	Roman Chamomile	Sandalwood	Spikenard	Rosemary
COMMAND®	Cassia	Peppermint	Oregano	Cilantro
COMMUNICATION®	Lavender	Spearmint	Lime	Cinnamon
COMPETITION®	Juniper Berry	Cassia	Siberian Fir	Thyme
CONNECTEDNESS®	Cedarwood	Frankincense	Marjoram	Oregano
CONSISTENCY®	Jasmine	Cedarwood	Patchouli	Bergamot
CONTEXT®	Copaiba	Frankincense	Siberian Fir	Clary Sage
DELIBERATIVE®	Rose	Arborvitae	Juniper Berry	Marjoram
DEVELOPER®	Lemongrass	Myrrh	Patchouli	Wintergreen
DISCIPLINE®	Cardamom	Neroli	Melaleuca	Petitgrain
EMPATHY®	Myrrh	Lime	Geranium	Oregano
FOCUS®	Vetiver	Cedarwood	Lemon	Rosemary
FUTURISTIC®	Clary Sage	Cypress	Geranium	Spikenard
HARMONY®	Petitgrain	Neroli	Coriander	Cassia

Talent Theme	Oil 1	Oil 2	Oil 3	Counterbalance
IDEATION®	Tangerine	Clary Sage	Juniper Berry	Vetiver
INCLUDER®	Melaleuca	Cedarwood	Frankincense	Clove
INDIVIDUALIZATION®	Black Pepper	Bergamot	Coriander	Cedarwood
INPUT®	Siberian Fir	Lavender	Rosemary	Clove
INTELLECTION®	Frankincense	Rosemary	Siberian Fir	Spearmint
LEARNER®	Melissa	Rosemary	Douglas Fir	Ginger
MAXIMIZER®	Patchouli	Copaiba	Fennel	Bergamot
POSITIVITY®	Ylang Ylang	Tangerine	Lime	Black Pepper
RELATOR®	Marjoram	Cedarwood	Coriander	Rosemary
RESPONSIBILITY®	Fennel	Ginger	Cardamom	Ylang Ylang
RESTORATIVE™	Basil	Geranium	Ylang Ylang	Thyme
SELF-ASSURANCE®	Bergamot	Grapefruit	Ginger	Wintergreen
SIGNIFICANCE®	Cinnamon	Spearmint	Frankincense	Oregano
STRATEGIC®	Clary Sage	Vetiver	Juniper Berry	Lemongrass
WOO®	Ylang Ylang	Jasmine	Spearmint	Grapefruit

BIBLIOGRAPHY

Asplund, Jim, James K. Harter, Sangeeta Agrawal, and Stephanie K. Plowman. 2015. *The Relationship Between Strengths-based Employee Development and Organizational Outcomes*. Washington, DC: Gallup®.

Bushdid, C., M. O. Magnasco, L. B. Vosshall, and A. Keller. 2014. "Humans Can Discriminate More Than 1 Trillion Olfactory Stimuli." *Science* 21: 1370–72.

Enlighten Alternative Healing, LLC. 2017. *Emotions and Essential Oils A Reference Guide for Emotional Healing*. 6th ed. Salt Lake City, Utah: Enlighten Alternative Healing, LLC.

NLP Anchoring. 2017. "Ken Ward's Mind Mastery Course." Accessed January 10. trans4mind.com/personal_development/mindMastery/anchoring.htm

NLP Secrets. 2017. "Anchoring: NLP Technique." Accessed January 10. www.nlp-secrets.com/nlp-technique-anchoring.php.

Rath, Tom. 2007. *Strengths Finder 2.0*. New York: Gallup Press.

Total Wellness Publishing. 2017. *The Essential Life: A Simple Guide to Living the Wellness Lifestyle*. 4th ed. Brownstown, MI: Total Wellness Publishing, LLC.

TO PURCHASE

To purchase *Anchor to Your Strengths*
in bulk for a discount, visit
www.anchortoyourstrengths.com.

To purchase essential oils, roller bottles,
and blend labels, visit
www.anchortoyourstrengths.com.

To discover your Top 5
CliftonStrengths®, please visit
www.gallupstrengthscenter.com.

ABOUT THE AUTHOR

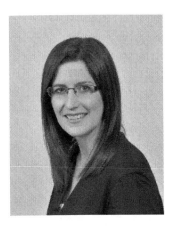

Melinda Brecheisen is an entrepreneur, business coach, mentor, and public speaker. She lives in the Bay Area of California with her husband, Jeremie, and their three children. She has been an ardent student of both CliftonStrengths® and essential oils for more than seven years. Her passion is to support others in becoming the best version of themselves so that they can make their own unique contributions to the world.

Made in the USA
Columbia, SC
06 February 2019